The Perfect Cookbook for Gestational Diabetes Patients

Manage Gestational Diabetes with
These 25 Recipes

By

Heston Brown

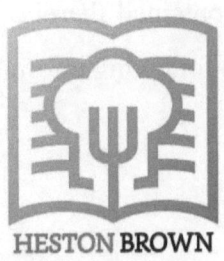

HESTON BROWN

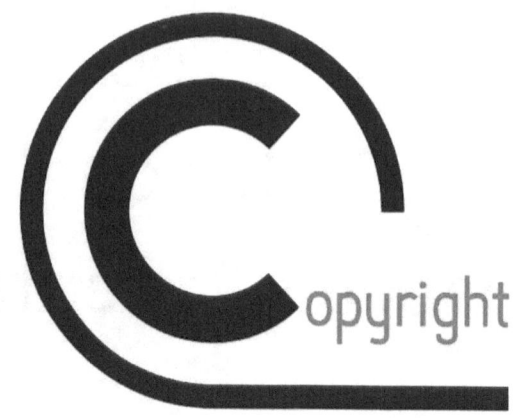

Copyright 2019 Heston Brown

Thank you so much for buying my book! I want to give you a special gift!

Receive a special gift as a thank you for buying my book. Now you will be able to benefit from free and discounted book offers that are sent directly to your inbox every week.

To subscribe simply fill in the box below with your details and start reaping the rewards! A new deal will arrive every day and reminders will be sent so you never miss out. Fill in the box below to subscribe and get started!

https://heston-brown.getresponsepages.com

Subscribe to our newsletter

Your Email >

Table of Contents

Chapter I - What Exactly Is Gestational Diabetes?

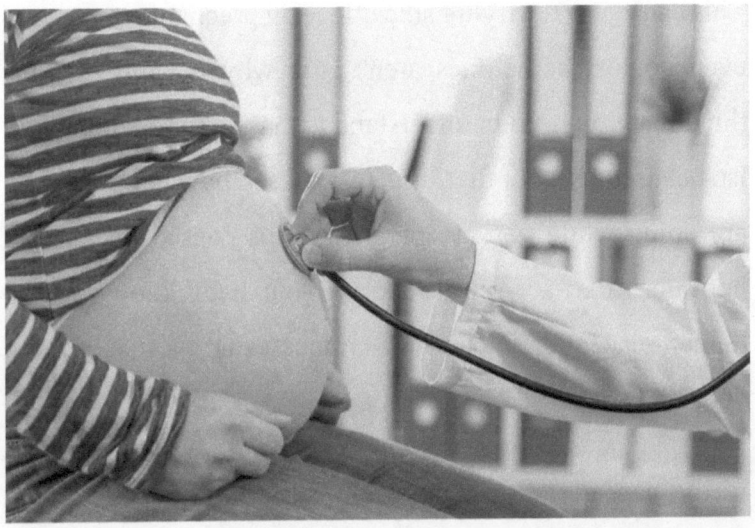

Before we get into the actual fun stuff of gestational recipes, we first must understand what gestational diabetes actually is. Technically it is known as insulin-dependent which means that the cells within your body aren't listening to the insulin signals that they are given. Because of this your pancreas will secrete insulin when it detects there's too much sugar in your blood and it will do this to give you excess blood sugar.

When your cells do not listen to these insulin signals anymore, your body will still continue to produce blood sugar and thus elevate your blood sugar levels in general.

This can cause terrifying side effects in pregnant women and even doctors sometimes aren't sure why it happens. One thing that you need to understand is that gestational diabetes isn't caused by your diet. It is just caused by what your cells are doing while you are pregnant. It is caused because of hormones that are released from your baby known as the human placental lactogen which messes up these signals in your body.

In the past gestational diabetes, while not really knowing how to deal with it, was scarier than it is today. In the past this type of diabetes usually would cause changes within both the maternal and Fetal environment, can cause complications during pregnancy and there was a high risk of emergency C-sections. However, today this is not the case as many people have found that by reducing your blood sugar levels you can help decrease all of these complications.

There are two primary ways that you can control your gestational diabetes. The first part will solely focus on you so you will need to make sure that your blood sugar levels are cut down so that you can be fine as your pregnancy carries on. The second part is going to be making sure that your baby is healthy and happy and his born that way.

XXXXXXXXXXXXXXXXXXXXXXXXXXXXXXXXXXXXXXXX

(1) Risk Factors of Gestational Diabetes

Now that you understand what gestational diabetes is, let's look at a few tests that you can have to make sure that you do or do not have this type of diabetes. It is always important to talk with your doctor about your risk factors and tests that can be done to ensure both you and your baby are kept healthy.

There are always a few warning flags that can lead a doctor to recommend you getting your blood sugar levels tested. While many of them can be obvious, here are a few risk factors that you may not necessarily know about.

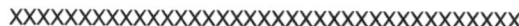

(2) Diabetes Runs in Your Family

If diabetes is prevalent within your family, then you may be at risk to developing gestational diabetes. This is because you have a genetic predisposition to developing it and you are more likely to develop it than somebody who doesn't. This is a huge factor and it is something worth getting tested for if this is the case.

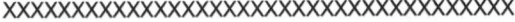

xxxxxxxxxxxxxxxxxxxxxxxxxxxxxxxxxxxxxxxxx

(3) Over the Age of Thirty

If you are having a baby over the age of 30, your risk for developing gestational diabetes is somewhat higher. You are at risk for a lot of conditions during your pregnancy including this type of diabetes. If you are over the age of 30 your doctor will automatically want to run a test to be on the safe side rather than take a risk you later on.

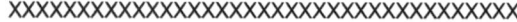

(4) Weight Issues

If you are a person who is overweight, this obesity can in fact increase the risk of developing gestational diabetes. However, keep in mind it is not a direct link.

xxxxxxxxxxxxxxxxxxxxxxxxxxxxxxxxxxxxxxxxx

(5) If You Come from an Ethnic Background

Most Caucasian women who become pregnant are not at risk to developing gestational diabetes. There are few groups out there that have a higher risk to developing it and if you come from an ethnic background this is something that you may need to be wary of. While this factor may not necessarily prompt your doctor to automatically send you for test, it can be one indication that you might be at risk for developing this type of diabetes.

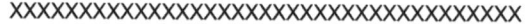

xxxxxxxxxxxxxxxxxxxxxxxxxxxxxxxxxxxxxx

(6) Previous Problems in Your Past pregnancies

If you have had a large baby in your past that was over 8 pounds or have suffered from a variety of miscarriages and stillbirths, a gestational diabetes test is one that your doctor will want to perform as soon as possible. It has been shown that have abnormalities within pregnancy can be linked to gestational diabetes so it is always better to get tested then be sorry for it later on.

xxxxxxxxxxxxxxxxxxxxxxxxxxxxxxxxxxxxxx

(7) Glucose in Your Urine

This is fair lease simple in terms of a symptom of gestational diabetes. When you go for your prenatal checkups you will always be asked to give a sample of your urine. If your doctors have found glucose in your urine they will automatically send you off to have a test done to see if you have gestational diabetes. However, keep in mind if you do have glucose in your urine it does not necessarily mean that you will be diagnosed with gestational diabetes.

XXXXXXXXXXXXXXXXXXXXXXXXXXXXXXXXXXXXXX

Chapter II - How to Test for Gestational Diabetes

If you have any of these risk factors that I have listed in the previous section, then most likely you will require to be tested for gestational diabetes. There a variety of different tests that you can have performed and most come in two different types. The first test will be a challenge test while the second test will be known as a tolerance test. If you are a woman that passes the first test, then you don't have anything to worry about. However, you may have to take a second test but could pass that as well. Regardless, here are the different types of tests that you will need to take if you are being tested for gestational diabetes.

XXXXXXXXXXXXXXXXXXXXXXXXXXXXXXXXXXXXXXXX

(1) The Tolerance Test

This type of test is usually done about 3 days after you have taken the first challenge test. During this test you can eat whatever you like, but you will have to fast for at least 12 hours before you get tested to make sure that your blood sugar level isn't high.

This type of test is also simple, except this time the syrup that you will be drinking contains 100 grams of glucose. It will follow same line as the other one, being tested after 1, two and three hours after you drink your sugar drink. If your blood sugar levels are higher than normal during these hours, then you have gestational diabetes.

XXXXXXXXXXXXXXXXXXXXXXXXXXXXXXXXXXXXX

(2) The Challenge Test

This test is pretty straightforward, and you don't really have to do anything on your part to prepare. All that you will have to do is drink a glucose syrup drink that has about 50 grams of glucose in it. Then all you have to do is sit around for an hour and have your blood drawn after. This blood draw will test to see how much sugar is in your blood after that hour. Sometimes you will have to wait 2 more hours and be tested every hour from then on.

If your blood sugar levels are normal, then after an hour it shouldn't be much above average. However, if your blood sugar levels are high even after that hour then most likely you have developed gestational diabetes. If you don't have that much blood sugar within your bloodstream, then you will be able to go home right after. However, if your blood sugar levels are high then there is a second test that you need to take in order to definitively know if you have gestational diabetes.

XXXXXXXXXXXXXXXXXXXXXXXXXXXXXXXXXXXXX

(3) The Hemoglobin Test

Another test that you will have is a hemoglobin test also known as glycosylated hemoglobin test or HbA1C. This test is done using your own blood, as you will be thoroughly tested throughout your pregnancy and will find high blood sugar within the cells of your hemoglobin. If your hemoglobin test is less than 6.5% then you are in the clear, but if it is higher than your doctor will most likely send you off to get more tests.

xxxxxxxxxxxxxxxxxxxxxxxxxxxxxxxxxxxxxxx

Chapter III - How Gestational Diabetes Can Affect Your Pregnancy

If you have gone through the various tests I have listed above and have come out positive with gestational diabetes, it is important for you to know about the potential risks and changes that can occur during your pregnancy. With today's modern medicine most of the time most mothers come out just fine through this initial period. However, it is always good to have a thorough understanding of how gestational diabetes can affect your pregnancy.

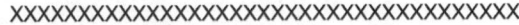

XXXXXXXXXXXXXXXXXXXXXXXXXXXXXXXXXXXXXXX

(1) Effects on the Mother

1. Infection

As a person suffering from gestational diabetes the first thing that you need to understand is that you are more prone to infection than any other person. This is because your immune system is already diminished so that it does not have an effect on your baby while you are carrying your baby to term. Because of this one of the infections that you are more susceptible to with gestational diabetes is urinary tract infections.

While this may not be a bad infection to deal with, most mothers may panic and this in turn can cause preterm labor. It also spreads very quickly if not treated by your doctor immediately. If you have the signs of a urinary tract infection which is usually a burning sensation whenever you use the bathroom or running to the bathroom very often, make sure that you talk to your doctor about what could possibly be happening.

XXXXXXXXXXXXXXXXXXXXXXXXXXXXXXXXXXXXX

2. Pre-Eclampsia

Gestational diabetes will also put you at risk to developing preeclampsia. This condition is known to cause hypertension which can then lead to complications around your liver and kidneys. It could also affect the blood flow to your baby. Preeclampsia is a very scary risk to deal with and since you are going to be tested a lot during your pregnancy your doctor will be able to have a handle on it before it gets out of hand.

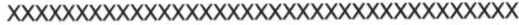

XXXXXXXXXXXXXXXXXXXXXXXXXXXXXXXXXXXXXXXX

3. Polyhydramnios

Another complication that can occur with gestational diabetes is known as polyhydramnios or swelling of the bump. The main issue here lies with amniotic fluid that your baby is swimming in. When this occurs the excess sugar within your body can lead into the baby's filter system and can sometimes get right into the amniotic fluid via your end. This can draw a lot of water from your body and diminish the amount of amniotic fluid available for your fetus.

This condition can lead to preterm labor and excessive bleeding after delivery. While it is not a common condition to suffer from, if you are a person who is suffering from unusual pain always ask your doctor to be safe than sorry.

xxxxxxxxxxxxxxxxxxxxxxxxxxxxxxxxxxxxx

4. Baby Growth

It is common knowledge that babies who get a lot of sugar tend to gain a lot of weight. When you suffer from gestational diabetes you will be giving your baby just that but more so than you should. This can lead to babies growing to be a large size and while this isn't a terrible thing it can complicate your overall delivery.

Larger babies tend to need small surgeries in order to get out and with a little assistance which can also increase the risk of complications after the surgery.

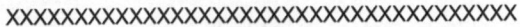

(2) Effects on the Baby

1. Spontaneous Abortions

In mothers who are diabetic there is an increased risk of developing congenital abnormalities in your baby. The main risk comes from the sugar that is in your bloodstream. The higher the sugar, the higher the risk is. One of the most common problems in mothers who suffer from high blood sugar levels is ventricular septal defect. This is a heart condition that can occur in fetuses, though it is fairly common and easily treatable. It can be checked for the moment your baby is born and only requires a simple surgery to fix.

XXXXXXXXXXXXXXXXXXXXXXXXXXXXXXXXXXXXX

2. Persistent Hyperglycemia

In the case of a mother who is suffering from gestational diabetes the pancreas of your baby may have to work a little harder to deal with the amount of glucose it is getting. This can lead to an excess of fat production and again cause problems around the heart and pancreas. This usually happens when your sugar level is too high and is not in control so this is something you need to heed your doctor's advice on.

While it is not a fatal problem, it is a problem that can be dealt with easily. Keep in mind this can lead to a very difficult labor but shouldn't have any long-lasting effects.

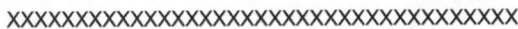

3. Post Birth Low Blood Sugar

Because of the fact that your baby will be dealing with high blood sugar levels this can lead to a production of large amounts of insulin. This can mean that when your baby is born it may have to adjust to no sugar being produced in the bloodstream. This can leave your baby to break down all of its own sugar way too quickly which could eventually lead to brain damage. However, after your baby is born this is something your baby's doctors and nurses when will closely monitor.

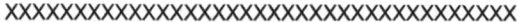

xxxxxxxxxxxxxxxxxxxxxxxxxxxxxxxxxxxxxx

4. May Have Breathing Issues

One final problem that may persist in your baby after they are born is that they are unable to breathe for short period of time. The main reason this happens is because your diabetes stops your baby from producing a liquid called surfactant which keeps your baby's lungs fully open and helps to make breathing much easier.

If this occurs your baby may have to stay in the hospital for a longer period of time, but should be able to recover from it fairly quickly.

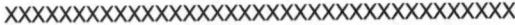

Chapter IV - Healthy Gestational Diabetes Recipes

xxxxxxxxxxxxxxxxxxxxxxxxxxxxxxxxxxxxxxxx

Recipe 1: Delicious Fish Kebabs and Potato Salad

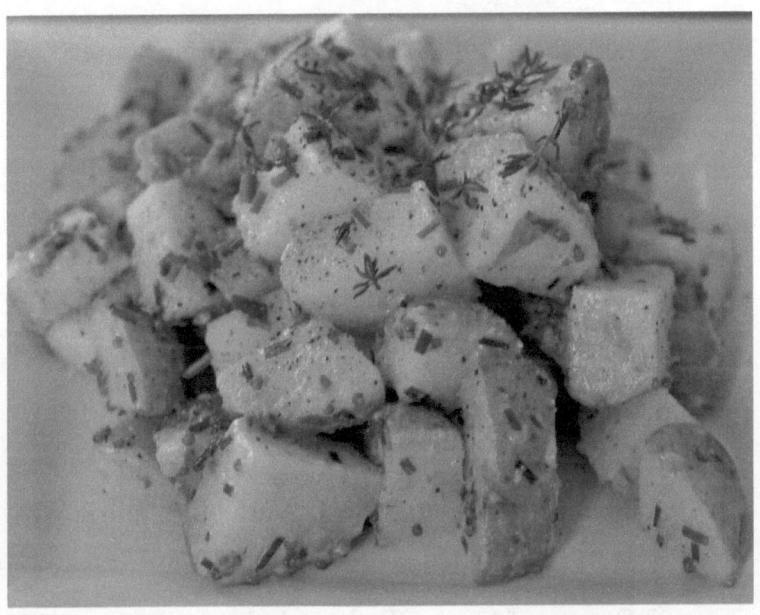

If you have been looking for a filling and delicious dish to make, this is one dish that I know you won't be able to resist. For the tastiest results I highly recommend marinating this dish in your fridge for as long as possible.

Yield: 4 Servings

Preparation Time: 20 Minutes

List of Ingredients:

- 1 ½ Pound of Fish Fillet, White in Color, Firm and Chopped Finely
- 2 tablespoons of Olive Oil, Extra Virgin Variety
- 1 Lemon, Large in Size, Rind and Juice Only
- ¼ Cup of Oregano, Fresh and Coarsely Chopped
- 2 Cloves of Garlic, Crushed
- ½ teaspoon of Cinnamon, Ground Variety
- Dash of Black Pepper, For Taste

Ingredients for Your Potato Salad:

- 2 Pounds of Potatoes, New Variety, Small in Size and Cut into Halves
- 3 Ounces of Yogurt, Plain and Low in Fat
- 1 Tablespoon of Mustard, Seeded Variety
- 1 Cucumber, Large in Size and Cut into Small Sized Pieces
- Some Green Veggies, Your Favorite Kind and for Serving

xxxxxxxxxxxxxxxxxxxxxxxxxxxxxxxxxxxxxxxxx

Instructions:

1. First thread your fish chunks onto your skewers. Place into a shallow ceramic bowl.

2. Please place your oil, lemon rind, fresh lemon juice, oregano, ground cinnamon and garlic into a large sized jar. Season with a dash of salt and pepper and shake well to combine.

3. Pour this marinade over your kebabs and toss thoroughly to combine.

4. Cover with some plastic wrap and allow to marinate for the next hour.

5. While your fish is marinating, bring a large sized pot of water to a boil. Once your water is boiling add in your potatoes and cook for the next 10 minutes or until firm to the touch. Remove from heat and drain.

6. Toss your potatoes with your cucumber, yogurt and mustard until evenly coated

7. Preheat a grill to high heat. Once it is hot enough grill your kebabs for the next 6 minutes.

8. Serve your kebabs with your fresh potato salad and enjoy.

Recipe 2: Savory Chicken Burritos

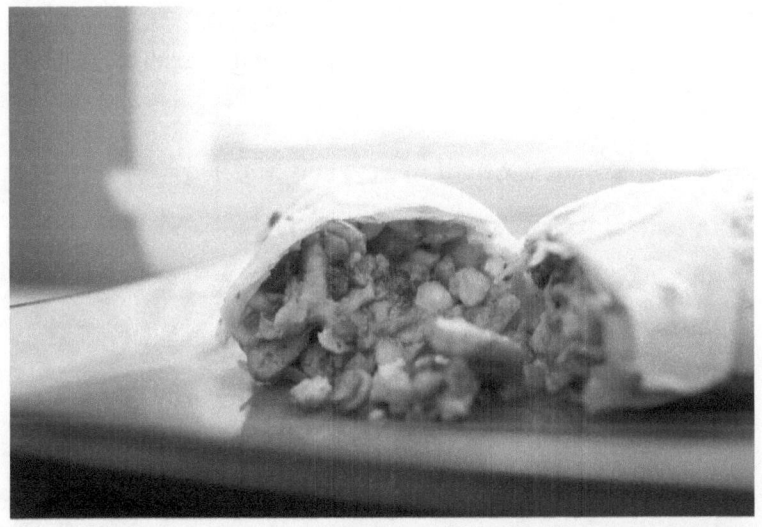

Need a dish to take along with you on the go? Then this is the perfect dish for you to make. It is an easy dish to make when you are feeling particularly lazy. For the best results I highly recommend allowing everybody top off these burritos with their favorite toppings.

Yield: 4 Servings

Preparation Time: 15 Minutes

List of Ingredients:

- 1 Pound of Chicken Breast, Thinly Sliced
- 1 ½ Tablespoon of Spice, Mexican Variety
- 2 Carrots, Fresh and Grated
- 1 Avocado, Small in Size and Mashed
- 1 Clove of Garlic, Crushed and Mixed with Some Avocado
- 1 Capsicum, Red in Color, Hulled and Sliced Thinly
- 1 Head of Lettuce, Butter Variety, Washed and Torn Roughly
- 1 Red Onion, Small in Size, cut into Halves and Thinly Sliced\
- 1 Bunch of Coriander, Chopped Roughly
- 2 Limes, Fresh and Cut into Quarters
- ½ Cup of Sour Cream, Light Variety
- 8 Pieces of Flat Bread, Low GI Variety

xxxxxxxxxxxxxxxxxxxxxxxxxxxxxxxxxxxxxxx

Instructions:

1. Place your chicken and Mexican spice into a large sized Ziploc bag. Shake thoroughly to coat.

2. Then heat up some oil in a large sized skillet placed over medium heat.

3. Once the oil is hot enough add in your chicken and cook for at least 5 to 8 minutes or until it is golden in color and fully cooked through.

4. Next arrange your remaining ingredients onto a large sized serving plate and serve your burritos according to each individual's preference. Enjoy.

Recipe 3: Classic Breakfast Porridge

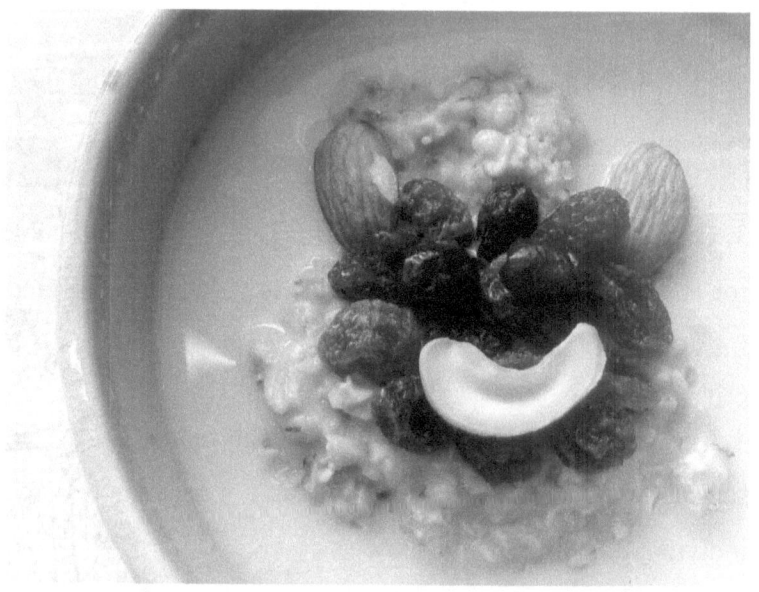

This is a great way to ensure you are getting your daily dose of carbohydrates while you are pregnant. It will help to keep you and your baby satisfied as well as help hold you over to your next meal.

Yield: 2 Servings

Preparation Time: 10 Minutes

Ingredients for Your Porridge:

- 1 Cup of Oats, Rolled Variety
- ½ teaspoon of Cinnamon, Ground Variety
- 2 ½ Cups of Water, Warm
- 1 Cup of Milk, Reduced in Fat

Ingredients for Your Fruit:

- 1 Apple, Small in Size and Finely Grated
- 1 Banana, Small in Size and Thinly Sliced
- ½ Cup of Berries, Fresh

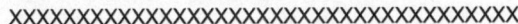

xxxxxxxxxxxxxxxxxxxxxxxxxxxxxxxxxxxxxxx

Instructions:

1. Place your oats, ground cinnamon and water into a small sized saucepan. Heat over low heat and stir constantly for the next 5 to 7 minutes.

2. Allow to simmer for another 5 minutes by adding in your remaining water.

3. Remove from heat.

4. Spoon at least half a cup of porridge into your serving bowls and serve with milk and your favorite kind of fruit. Sprinkle your cinnamon as garnish and enjoy.

Recipe 4: Pesto Smothered Pasta with Chicken

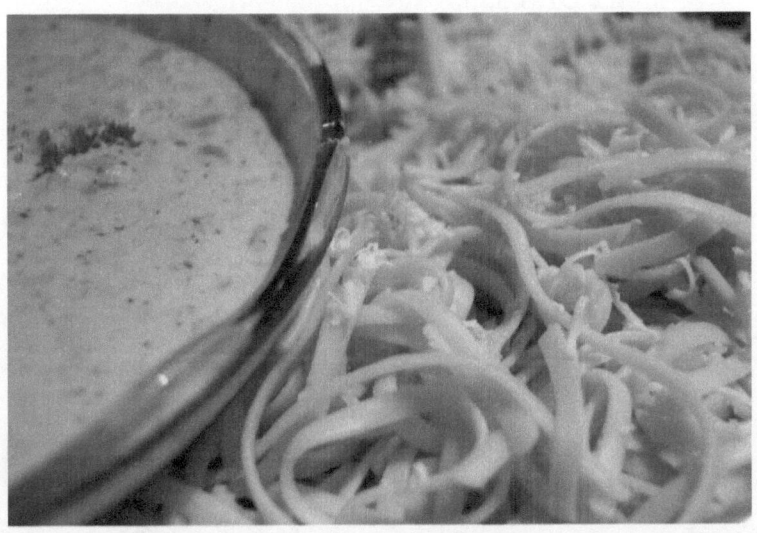

If you are a huge fan of both pasta and chicken, then this is the perfect dish for you to make. It makes for a simple late night dinner to enjoy and that you can make if you want to impress your friends and family.

Yield: 4 Servings

Preparation Time: 15 Minutes

List of Ingredients:

- 2 Chicken Breasts, Skinless and Boneless Variety
- Some Olive Oil, Extra Virgin Variety
- ½ Pound of Green Beans, Fresh and Trimmed
- ½ Pound of Cherry Tomatoes, Cut into Quarters
- 1 Pound of Pasta, Fettucine Variety and Fully Cooked

Ingredients for Your Pesto:

- 2 Cloves of Garlic, Peeled and Crushed
- 1 Bunch of Basil, Fresh and Torn Roughly
- 1 Lemon, Zest and Juice Only
- 4 Tablespoon of Parmesan Cheese, Freshly Grated
- 1 Tablespoon of Olive Oil, Extra Virgin Variety
- Dash of Salt and Pepper, For Taste

xxxxxxxxxxxxxxxxxxxxxxxxxxxxxxxxxxxxx

Instructions:

1. The first thing that you will want to do is combine all of your ingredients for your pesto into a large sized bowl. Stir thoroughly using a hand blender until evenly mixed. Set aside for later use.

2. Next cook your pasta according to the directions on the package. Once your pasta is cooked add to your pesto and stir to thoroughly combine. Cover and set aside for later use.

3. Then blanch your green beans according to your preference.

4. Season your chicken fillets with some salt and pepper.

5. Add a large sized skillet placed over medium heat. Add in your oil and once your oil is hot enough add your chicken fillet and cook for at least 5 to 8 minutes on each side or until fully cooked through.

6. Add in your tomatoes and continue to cook for the next 5 minutes before removing from heat.

7. Serve while still piping hot and enjoy.

Recipe 5: Early Morning Frittata

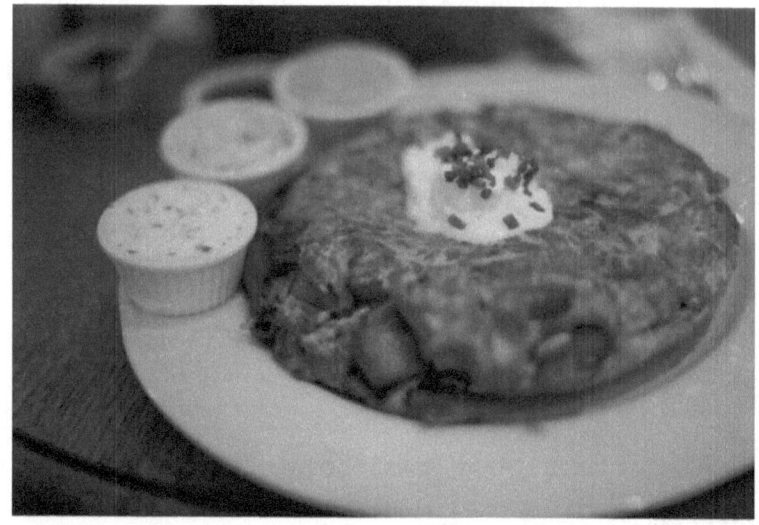

Here is yet another breakfast recipe to make if you are looking for something more on the filling side. It makes plenty of food for one large breakfast, so it is enough to serve a large group of people along with yourself.

Yield: 2 Servings

Preparation Time: 40 Minutes

List of Ingredients:

- 1 Tablespoon of Oil, Light and Cooking Variety
- ½ of a Leek, Sliced Thinly and Washed
- ½ of a Red Onion, Chopped Finely
- 7 Ounces of Potatoes, New Variety, Small in Size, Peeled and Thinly Sliced
- 1 Zucchini, Large in Size and Sliced into Rounds
- 4 Eggs, Large in Size and Beaten Lightly
- 3 Ounces of Ricotta Cheese, Reduced in Fat
- 1 to 2 Slices of Toast, Whole Grain Variety

xxxxxxxxxxxxxxxxxxxxxxxxxxxxxxxxxxxxxxx

Instructions:

1. The first thing that you will want to do is preheat your oven to 425 degrees.

2. While your oven is heating up heat some oil over medium heat in a small sized skillet. Once the oil add in your leeks, onions and potatoes into it. Season with a dash of pepper and cook until your leeks and onions are soft to the touch. This should take at least 5 minutes.

3. After this time add in your zucchini and stir well to combine.

4. Add in your eggs and ricotta next and stir thoroughly to combine.

5. Continue to cook over medium heat for the next 2 to 3 minutes or until your eggs are fully cooked through. This should take at least 10 to 15 minutes.

6. Continue to cook over low heat for the next 10 minutes to ensure it fluffs up nicely.

7. Remove from heat, flip onto a plate and serve whenever you are ready. Enjoy.

Recipe 6: San Choy Bau

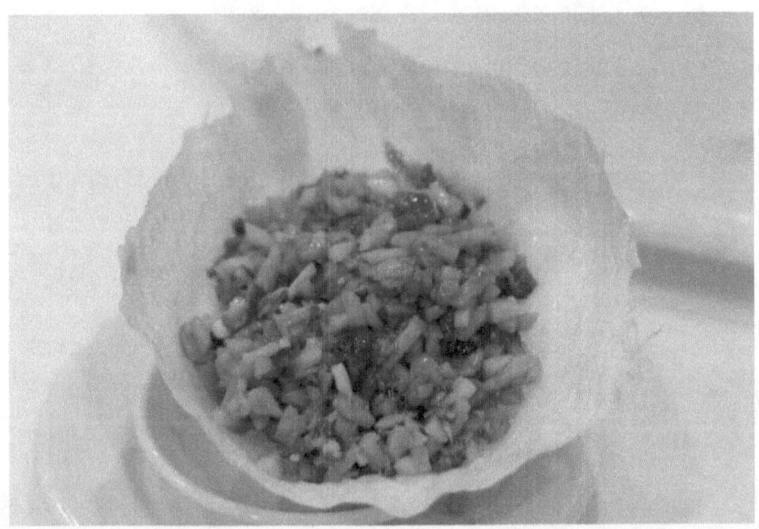

If you are looking for an exotic dish, then this is the perfect dish for you to make. While there are a lot of ingredients in this dish, it is so delicious, it is well worth the effort to making it.

Yield: 4 Servings

Preparation Time: 12 Minutes

List of Ingredients:

- ¾ Tablespoon of Oil, Sesame Variety
- ¾ Tablespoon of Oil, Cooking Variety
- 10 ½ Ounce of Pork, Crumbled
- 1 Tablespoon of Ginger, Fresh and Finely Grated
- 2 Cloves of Garlic, Finely Chopped
- 5/3 Ounces of Mushrooms, Button Variety and Finely Chopped
- 1 Red Chili, Fresh, Seeded and Chopped Finely
- 1, 5 Ounce Can of Chestnuts, Water Variety, Drained and Chopped Finely
- 3 Onions, Spring Variety and Finely Chopped
- 1 Ounce of Noodles, Vermicelli Variety and Fully Cooked
- 1 Carrot, Fresh, Large in Size and Grated
- 1 Zucchini, Large in Size and Grated
- 3 tablespoons of Soy Sauce, Reduced in Sodium
- 1 Lime, Juice Variety
- 2 tablespoons of Vinegar, Rice Wine Variety
- ½ Cup of Coriander Leaves, Roughly Chopped
- 4 Leaves of Iceberg Lettice, Large in Size
- Some Sesame Seeds, Toasted Variety and for Serving

XX

Instructions:

1. First heat up your oils in a large sized wok placed over low to medium heat. Once the oil is hot enough add in your tofu and cook until brown in color.

2. Add in your ginger, garlic, mushrooms and chili. Add in your chestnuts, onions, noodles, carrot and zucchini. Stir well to thoroughly combine.

3. Add in your fresh lime juice, vinegar and tamari. Stir again to combine.

4. Remove from heat and add in your coriander leaves. Toss thoroughly to combine.

5. Serve with a topping of your toasted sesame seeds and leaves of lettuce. Serve whenever you are reach

Recipe 7: Tasty Bircher Muesli

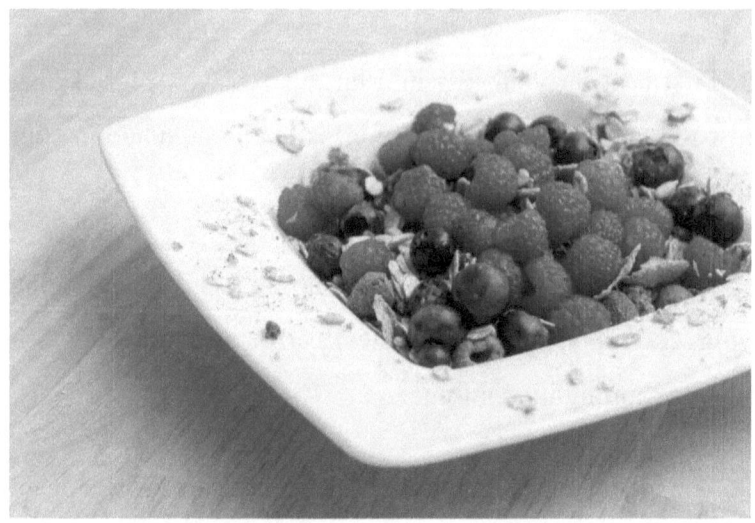

This is one dish that can help you to control your blood sugar levels throughout the entire day. While there are millions of recipes out there similar to this one, none are as delicious as this one.

Yield: 2 Servings

Preparation Time: 6 to 8 Servings

List of Ingredients:

- 3 Ounces of Oats, Rolled Variety
- 5 Ounces of Milk, Reduced in Fat
- 1 Orange, Small in Size and Rind Only
- 5 Ounces of Orange Juice, Fresh
- 5 Ounces of Water
- 1 Ounce of Almond Meal
- 2 teaspoons of Cinnamon, Ground Variety
- 2 tablespoons of Sesame Seeds, Toasted
- 1 Cup of Blueberries, Fresh

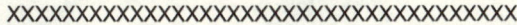

xxxxxxxxxxxxxxxxxxxxxxxxxxxxxxxxxxxxxxx

Instructions:

1. First combine your milk, fresh orange juice, water, almond, ground cinnamon, toasted sesame seeds, oats and fresh orange rind in a large sized bowl. Stir thoroughly until combined.

2. Cover with some plastic wrap and place into your fridge to chill for the next 6 to 8 hours.

3. After this time remove and stir well.

4. Top off with your blueberries and serve right away.

Recipe 8: Savory Curried Chicken with Beans and Currants

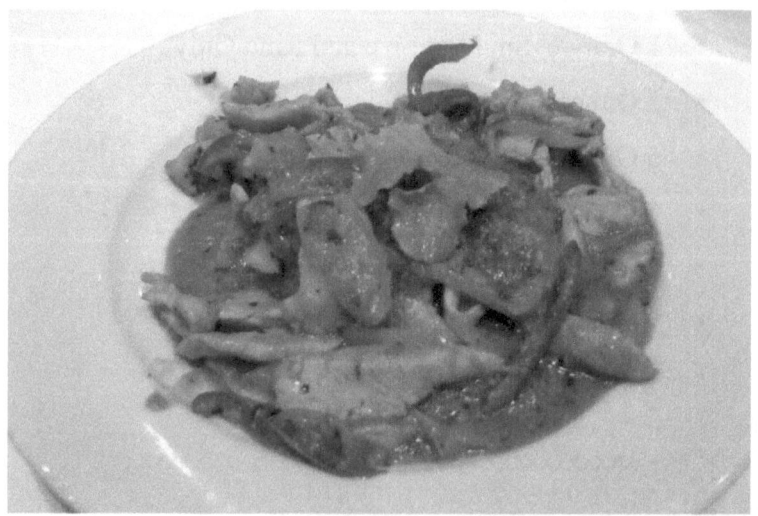

This is one curried chicken recipe that will certainly leave you wanting more. It makes for a delicious and easy dinner recipe that you can make for your entire family. This gestational diabetes friendly recipe is so savory, even the pickiest of eaters won't be able to resist it.

Yield: 4 Servings

Preparation Time: 15 Minutes

List of Ingredients:

- Some Cooking Spray
- 1 Brown Onion, Large in Size and Chopped Finely
- 2 to 3 Cloves of Garlic, Crushed
- 1 ½ Pounds of Chicken Breasts, Trimmed and Cut into Strips
- 2 tablespoons of Curry Powder
- 12 ½ Ounces of Milk, Skim and Evaporated Variety
- 1 Tablespoon of Coconut, Essence Variety
- 4 Tablespoon of Raisins, Your Favorite Kind
- 13 Ounces of Green Beans, Trimmed and Cut into Thirds
- 2 Cups of Rice, Fully Cooked and Low GI Variety
- Dash of Coriander, For Serving
- Dash of Cilantro, For Serving
- 2 Cucumbers, Peeled and Sliced Thoroughly

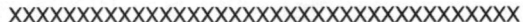

xxxxxxxxxxxxxxxxxxxxxxxxxxxxxxxxxxxxxxxx

Instructions:

1. Heat some oil in a large sized skillet placed over low heat. Once the oil is hot enough add in your onions and cook until they are translucent.

2. Then turn up the heat to medium and add in your chicken and garlic. Cook for the next 10 to 15 minutes or until your chicken is golden in color.

3. Add in your powder curry and stir well to combine. Continue to cook until fragrant.

4. Reduce the heat to low and add in your milk, currants and coconut.

5. Allow to simmer for the next 5 minutes before adding in your green beans.

6. Continue to simmer for another 5 to 10 minutes before removing from heat.

7. Serve your rice with a topping of curry, cilantro and coriander. Serve with a side of fresh cucumber and enjoy whenever you are ready.

Recipe 9: Delicious Baked Eggs with Tomato and Spinach

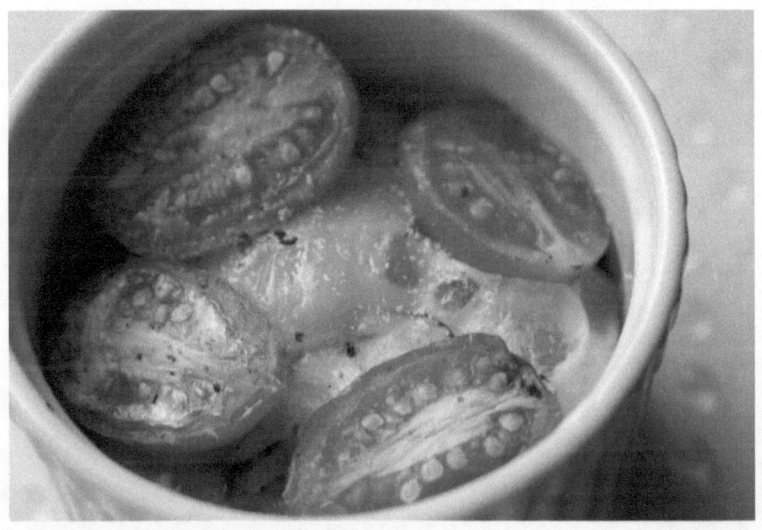

If you are looking for a more classy and delicious dish to enjoy every morning, this is one dish that you need to try to make for yourself. This dish is easy to make and can be easily adapted to best fit your needs.

Yield: 2 Servings

Preparation Time: 20 Minutes

List of Ingredients:

- Some Ramekins, Generously Greased
- 4 Eggs, Large in Size
- 2.5 Ounces of Cherry Tomatoes, Cut into Halves
- 1 ½ Tablespoon of Parmesan Cheese Freshly Grated
- 2.5 Ounce of Spinach Leaves, Baby Variety
- 4 Mushrooms, Large in Size and Thinly Sliced
- 1 to 2 Slices of Toast, Wholegrain Variety

xxxxxxxxxxxxxxxxxxxxxxxxxxxxxxxxxxxxxxx

Instructions:

1. The first thing that you will want to do is preheat your oven to 400 degrees. While your oven is heating up grease your ramekins with a generous amount of cooking spray.

2. Then use a medium sized skillet and add in some oil. Heat over medium heat and once it is hot enough add in your tomatoes and mushrooms and cook until brown in color.

3. Add in your spinach leaves and continue to cook while tossing for the next 1 to 2 minutes.

4. Remove from heat.

5. Spoon half of your mixture into each ramekin.

6. Crack your eggs over the top and sprinkle your cheese over the top. Season with some pepper.

7. Place into your oven to bake for the next 15 minutes or until your eggs are completely set.

8. Remove and serve with some toast and enjoy.

Recipe 10: Lemon and Thyme Roasted Chicken

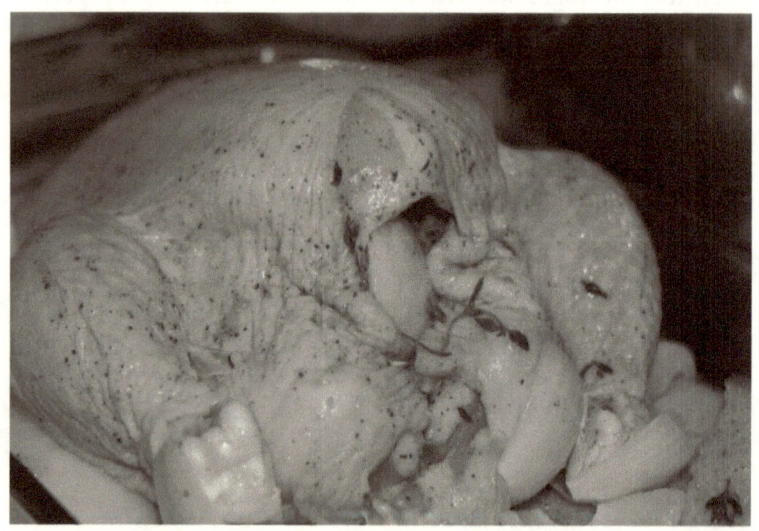

If you are looking for a range free chicken dish to enjoy, then this is the perfect dish for you to make. It is so delicious I can guarantee that you will want to make it over and over again.

Yield: 4 Servings

Preparation Time: 1 Hour and 15 Minutes

List of Ingredients:

- Some Cooking Spray
- 4 ½ Pounds of Chicken, Whole, Free Range Variety, Rinsed and Dried
- 1 Bunch of Thyme, Fresh, Washed and Dry
- 1 Lemon, Cut into Quarters
- ½ a Head of Garlic, Unpeeled and Separated
- 4 Carrots, Cut into Halves
- 1 ¾ Pounds of Potato, Washed, Peeled and Cut into Quarters
- Some Green Vegetables, Your Favorite Kind and for Serving

xxxxxxxxxxxxxxxxxxxxxxxxxxxxxxxxxxxxxxxx

Instructions:

1. The first thing that you will want to do is preheat your oven to 350 degrees.

2. While your oven is heating up wash your chicken under some cold running water and pat dry with a paper towel. Place into a large sized baking dish.

3. Fill the inside cavity of your chicken with your fresh thyme and tie the legs of the chicken together with some string.

4. Spray your chicken with some cooking spray and season the outside with some salt and pepper.

5. Around the chicken add in your fresh lemon, garlic, carrots and potatoes. Spray again with some cooking spray.

6. Place into your oven to bake for the next 1 ½ hours or until thoroughly cooked through.

7. Remove from oven and allow to cool slightly for at least 5 minutes before serving.

Recipe 11: Early Morning Breakfast Cups

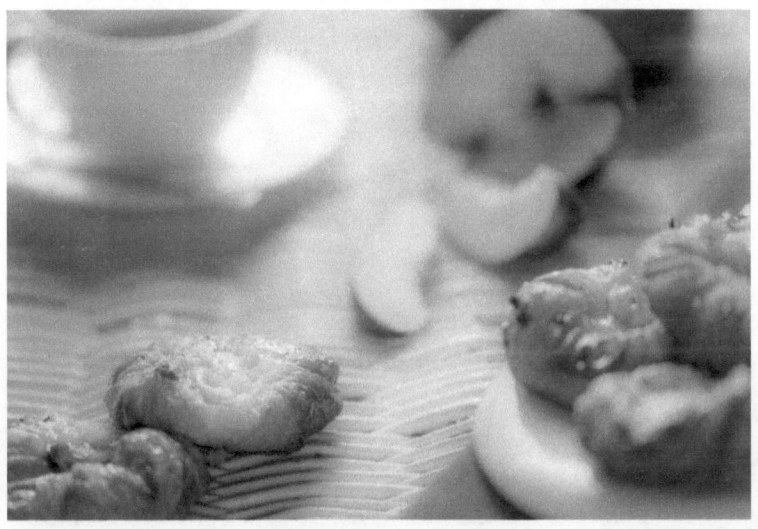

If you need an early morning dish to take along with you to your next doctor's appointment, then this is the perfect dish for you. These breakfast cups are incredibly delicious to make and make for the ultimate brunch picnic treat.

Yield: 4 Servings

Preparation Time: 15 Minutes

List of Ingredients:

- 6 Eggs, Large in Size and Beaten Lightly
- ¼ Cup of Parmesan Cheese, Freshly Grated
- 4 Asparagus Spears, Blanched and Cut into Small Pieces

xxxxxxxxxxxxxxxxxxxxxxxxxxxxxxxxxxxx

Instructions:

1. The first thing that you will want to do is preheat your oven to 400 degrees.

2. Then whisk your eggs into the cups of your muffin pan.

3. Evenly distribute you're your chopped asparagus evenly among your cups.

4. Sprinkle your cheese over the top.

5. Place into your oven to bake for the next 10 to 12 minutes or until your eggs are completely cooked and are fluffy in texture.

6. Remove and serve right away.

Recipe 12: Tarragon Style Roasted Fish

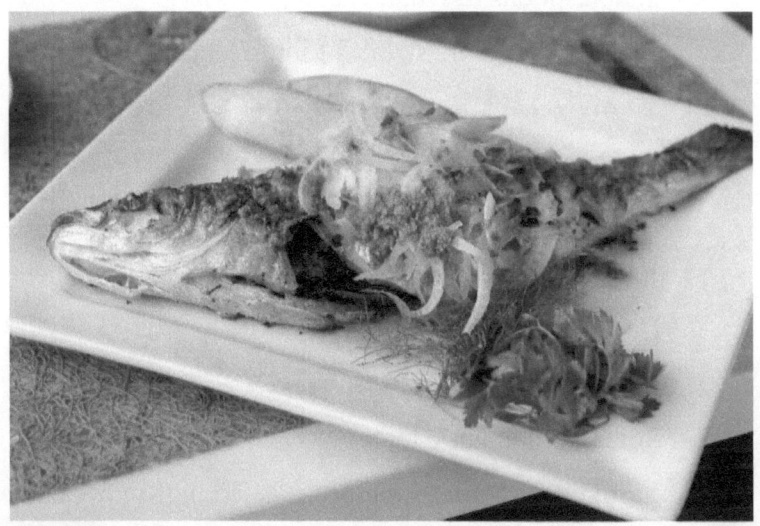

If you are a huge fan of fish, then this is one dish you are going to want to try making for yourself. It is incredibly easy to make and will help leave you feeling satisfied for the rest of the day.

Yield: 4 Servings

Preparation Time: 35 Minutes

List of Ingredients:

- 1 Whole Fish, Large in Size and Cleaned
- 2 tablespoons of Oil, Vegetable Variety
- 2 Leeks, Large in Size, Cut into Quarters and Sliced Thinly
- 2 Cloves of Garlic, Finely Sliced
- 1 Lemon, Large in Size and Juice Only
- 1 Lemon, Rind and Sliced into Small Sized Rounds
- Dash of Salt and Pepper, For Taste
- ½ Cup of Tarragon, Fresh
- Some Parchment Paper
- 1 Pound of Sweet Potatoes, Peeled, cut into Cubes and Roasted
- 1, 13 Ounce Can of Lentils, Drained and Rinsed
- Some Green Salad, For Serving

xxxxxxxxxxxxxxxxxxxxxxxxxxxxxxxxxxxxxxx

Instructions:

1. The first thing that you will want to do is preheat your oven to 350 degrees.

2. While your oven is heating up heat up some olive oil in a large sized skillet placed over low to medium heat. Once the oil is hot enough add in your leeks and garlic. Cook for at least 10 minutes or until they are soft to the touch.

3. Remove half of this mixture and set aside for your fish.

4. Remove your skillet from heat and add in your fresh lemon juice and rind. Season with some salt and pepper and stir to combine.

5. Next line a baking dish with some parchment paper.

6. Make 2 to 3 slashed within the surface of your fish. Brush it with a generous amount of oil and place into your baking dish. Spoon your leek mixture into these slashes and place your fresh lemon rounds around the outside of your fish. Season with some black pepper.

7. Fold the sides of the parchment paper to cover your fish and tuck the corners underneath.

8. Place into your oven to bake for the next 25 minutes.

9. After this time add in your oiled sweet potatoes into a small sized baking dish and place into your oven to bake along with your fish. Cook until it is tender to the touch.

10. When both are cooked combine your lentils with your remaining leek mixture. Season with a dash of salt and pepper.

11. Serve your fish with your sweet potatoes and lentil mixture on top of it. Serve while warm and enjoy.

Recipe 13: Classic French Toast

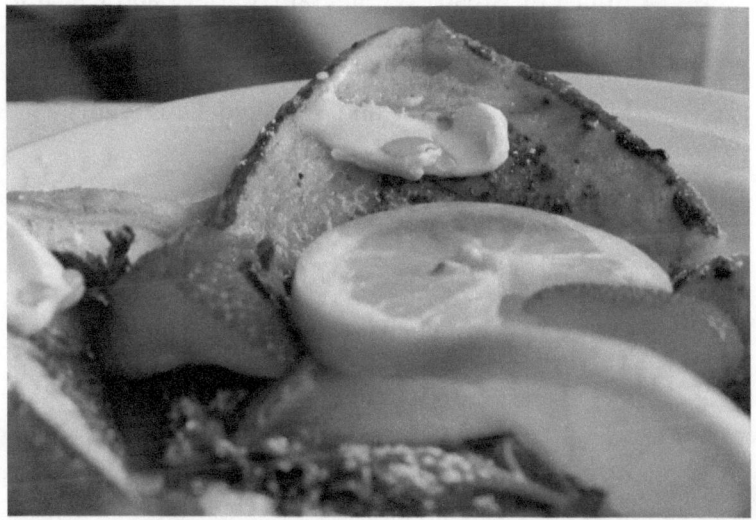

Are you a fan of classic French Toast? If so, then this is the perfect dish for you to make. The best part about this dish that it makes for a tasty breakfast meal that the entire family can easily enjoy.

Yield: 2 Servings

Preparation Time: 10 Minutes

List of Ingredients:

- 4 Slices of Bread, Wholegrain Variety and Cut into Halves
- 2 Eggs, Large in Size and Whisked Thoroughly
- ½ Cup of Milk, Low in Fat
- Some Cooking Spray
- 9 Ounces of Ricotta Cheese, Low in Fat
- 9 Ounces of Strawberries, Fresh and Thinly Sliced
- Dash of Cinnamon, Ground Variety and for Serving

xxxxxxxxxxxxxxxxxxxxxxxxxxxxxxxxxxxxxxx

Instructions:

1. Place your milk a small sized bowl and add in your whisked egg in another small sized bowl. Set aside for later use.

2. Next spray a large sized pan with some cooking oil and place over medium to high heat.

3. Dip a slice of bread into your milk first and then egg. Transfer your bread straight to your frypan. Repeat until all of your slices of bread have been used.

4. Cook for the next 2 to 3 minutes on each side of until golden in color.

5. Serve your French toast with a dollop of your ricotta cheese, strawberries and a dash of cinnamon for garnish. Enjoy.

Recipe 14: Peach Style Chicken Salad

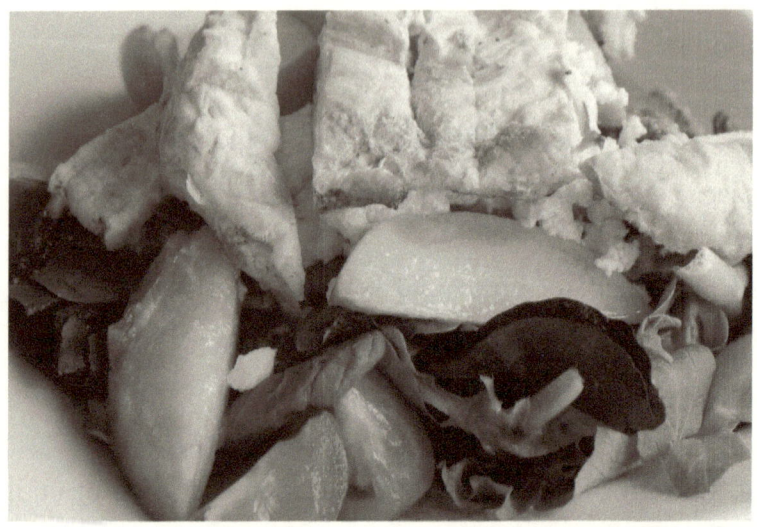

Here is a refreshing summer time salad that will become a sensational hit in your household. It is creamy in consistency, sweet tasty variety and slightly salted, making for a great tasting dish you are going to fall in love with.

Yield: 4 Servings

Preparation Time: 35 Minutes

List of Ingredients:

- 4 Chicken Fillets
- Some Cooking Spray
- 3 tablespoons of Vinegar, Balsamic Variety
- 13 Ounces of Potatoes, New Variety, Small in Size and Quartered
- 5 Ounces of Yogurt, Greek and Low-Fat Variety
- ½ Cup of Shallots, Finely Chopped
- 1 Orange, Small in Size, Zest and Juice Only
- 3 Tomatoes, Medium in Size, Trimmed and Cut into Quarters
- 1.3 Pounds of Peaches, Hulled and Cut into Quarters
- 1 Cucumber, Large in Size, Peeled, Halves and Finely Chopped
- 1/3 Cup of Mint Leaves, Fresh and Roughly Chopped
- 7 Ounces of Spinach Leaves, Roughly Torn

xxxxxxxxxxxxxxxxxxxxxxxxxxxxxxxxxxxxxx

Instructions:

1. Bring a large sized pot of water to a boil. Once your water is boiling add in your potatoes and cook for the next 10 minutes or until cooked. Remove, drain and set aside for later use.

2. Then grease a frying pan with some cooking spray. Place over medium to high heat.

3. Season both sides of your chicken with some salt and pepper. Place into pan to cook for at least 5 to 10 minutes or until fully cooked through.

4. Increase the heat to high and add in your vinegar. Cook until it slightly caramelizes.

5. After this time remove and allow to rest for at least 5 minutes before slicing.

6. Add your yogurt into your pan along with your shallots, fresh orange juice and zest. Stir thoroughly to combine. Season if you wish.

7. Use a large sized mixing bowl and add in your tomatoes, cucumber, peaches, fresh mint and cooked potatoes. Add in your yogurt dressing and toss to combine.

8. Add in your salad leaves and fold gently to mix.

9. Divide up your salad among your serving plates and top off with your cooked chicken. Serve right away and enjoy.

Recipe 15: Hearty Bacon, Lettuce, Tomato and Egg Sandwich

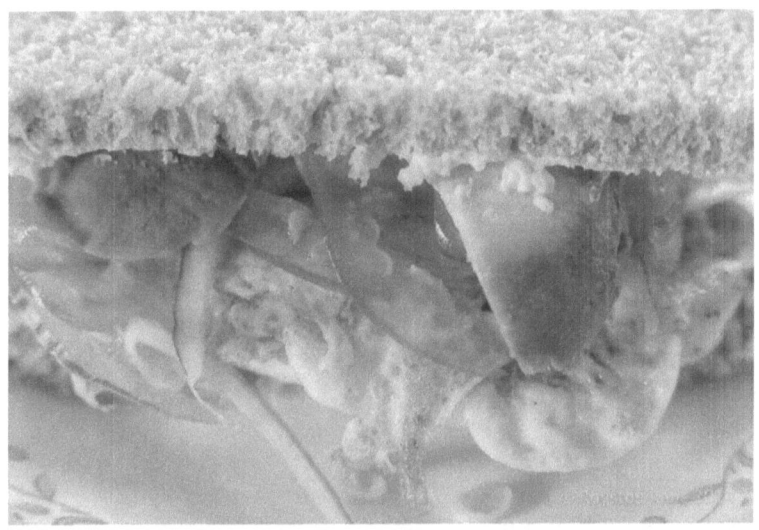

This is a delicious sandwich recipe that you can make if you are looking for a versatile dish that you can enjoy for breakfast or lunch. Regardless of when you serve it, I know you won't be able to get enough of it.

Yield: 2 Servings

Preparation Time: 7 Minutes

List of Ingredients:

- 4 Slices of Bread, Wholegrain Variety and Toasted Lightly
- 4 Rashers of Bacon, Trimmed and Low in Fat
- 4 Eggs, Large in Size
- 2 Tomatoes, Fresh and Thinly Sliced
- 1 Head of Lettuce, Leaves Separated and Baby Variety
- Some Chili Sauce, Your Favorite Kind

xxxxxxxxxxxxxxxxxxxxxxxxxxxxxxxxxxxxxx

Instructions:

1. The first thing that you are going to want to do is grill your bacon in a frying pan until completely cooked. Transfer into a large sized plate lined with paper towels to drain.

2. Then fry your eggs until completely cooked and toast your bread at the same time.

3. Next assemble your sandwich according to your preference, making sure your eggs and bacon are warm to the touch.

4. Serve your dish with some dill pickles and enjoy right away.

Recipe 16: Saffron Style Couscous Salad

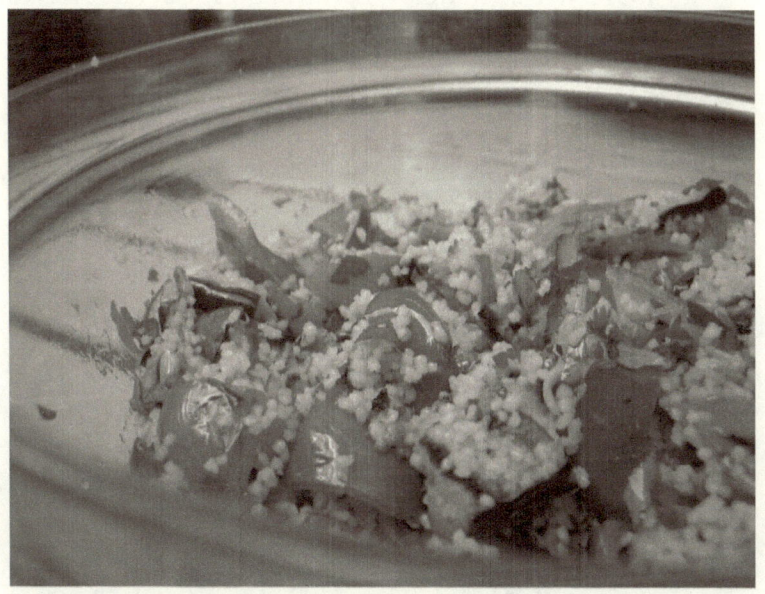

Here is yet another delicious and filling salad that I know you are going to love it. For the tastiest results I highly recommend serving this dish with some canned tuna to make a meal that you won't forget.

Yield: 4 Servings

Preparation Time: 15 Minutes

List of Ingredients:

- 1 Tablespoon of Olive Oil, Extra Virgin Variety
- 1 Onion, Red in Color, Large in Size, Cut into Halves and Sliced Thinly
- 2 tablespoons of tomato Paste
- 1 teaspoon of Cumin, Ground
- 1 teaspoon of Coriander
- 1 teaspoon of Cinnamon, Ground Variety
- ¼ teaspoon of Saffron Threads, Soaked in Water
- 1 Cup of Couscous, Fully Cooked
- 1 Capsicum, Red in Color and Sliced thinly
- 2 Tomatoes, Fresh and Finely Diced
- 6 Olives, Kalamata Variety and Thinly Sliced
- ½ Cup of Parsley, Flat Leaf Variety and Chopped Roughly
- ½ Cup of Orange Juice, Fresh and Squeezed
- 1 Lemon, Small in Size and Zested
- 7 Ounces of Yogurt, Low Fat Variety and Greek Variety
- 4 Pieces of Flat Bread, Mountain Bread Variety

xxxxxxxxxxxxxxxxxxxxxxxxxxxxxxxxxxxxxxxx

Instructions:

1. The first thing that you will want to do is cook your couscous according to the directions on the package.

2. Then heat up some olive oil in a large sized saucepan placed over medium heat. Once your oil is hot enough add in your onions and cook for the next 8 to 10 minutes or until translucent.

3. Add in your tomato paste, cumin, coriander and ground cinnamon. Stir to thoroughly combine.

4. Continue to cook for the next 3 to 4 minutes or until your spices are fragrant.

5. Add your saffron with the water and cooked couscous. Stir thoroughly to combine.

6. Add in your capsicum, olives, fresh tomatoes, chopped parsley, fresh orange juice and lemon zest. Stir well to combine.

7. Remove from heat and serve whenever you are ready.

Recipe 17: Creamy Potato Salad

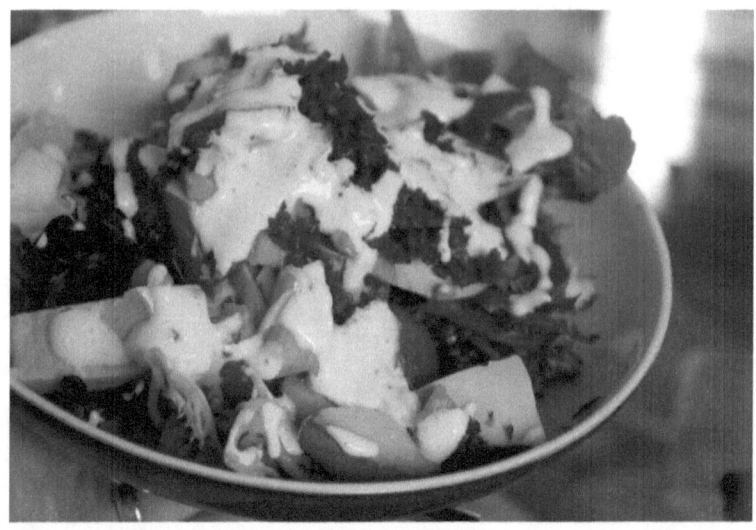

If you are looking for a dish that you can bring to your next family picnic, this is the perfect dish for you. Best of all you can utilize this healthy gestational diabetes recipe that you can easily turn into a meal.

Yield: 4 Servings

Preparation Time: 15 Minutes

List of Ingredients:

- 2 Pounds of Potatoes, New Variety, Small in Size and Cut into Halves
- 3 Ounces of Yogurt, Plain and Low in Fat
- 1 Tablespoon of Mustard, Seeded Variety
- 1 Cucumber, Large in Size and Cut into Small Sized Pieces
- Dash of Salt and Pepper, For Taste

xxxxxxxxxxxxxxxxxxxxxxxxxxxxxxxxxxxxxx

Instructions:

1. First bring a large sized pot of water to a boil. Once your water is boiling add in your potatoes and boil for at least 10 minutes or until firm to the touch. Once firm drain and allow to cool completely.

2. Once your potatoes are cooled to the touch add to a large sized bowl.

3. Add in your cucumber, yogurt and muster. Season with a dash of salt and pepper for taste and toss thoroughly to combine. Serve right away and enjoy.

Recipe 18: Healthy Poached Chicken Salad

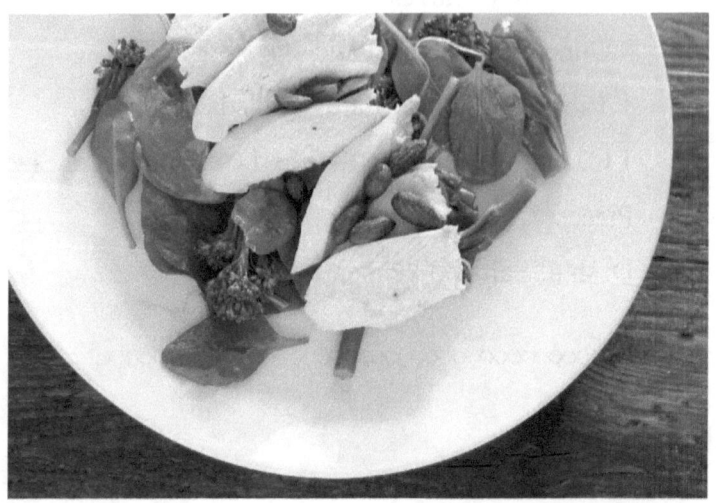

When it comes to this recipe, it will certainly get you excited about cooking with gestational diabetes. Feel free to make this dish using other veggies instead of green beans such as broccoli, spinach or lettuce. Either way I know you are going to love it.

Yield: 2 Servings

Preparation Time: 25 Minutes

List of Ingredients:

- 1 to 2 Cups of Stock, Chicken Variety
- 2 Chicken Breasts, Medium in Size and Cut into Halves
- 8 Ounces of Green Beans, Trimmed and Cut into Quarters
- 1, 13 Ounce Can of Beans, Cannellini Variety, Rinsed and Drained
- ¼ Cup of Mint, Roughly Torn
- ½ Cup of Parsley, roughly torn
- 1 Cup of Salad Greens, Your Favorite Kind
- 1 Tablespoon of Mustard, Honey Seed Variety
- 1 Lemon, Small in Size, Rind and Juice Only
- 1 tablespoon of Olive Oil, Extra Virgin Variety
- 1 Clove of Garlic, Crushed
- 1 teaspoon of Mint, Finely Chopped

xxxxxxxxxxxxxxxxxxxxxxxxxxxxxxxxxxxxxxx

Instructions:

1. The first thing that you will want to do is bring your chicken stock to a boil in a large sized saucepan. Once boiling reduce the heat to low.

2. Add in your chicken breasts and allow to simmer for the next 15 minutes. After this time remove your chicken and set aside.

3. Finely shred your chicken using two forks and place into a large sized mixing bowl.

4. Next bring a small sized saucepan filled with water to a boil. Once boiling blanch your beans for at least 2 to 3 minutes. After this time remove from heat and rinse with some cold water. Drain and set aside for later use.

5. Then make your dressing. To do this combine your fresh lemon juice, mustard, rind, chopped garlic, mint and olive oil.

6. Season with some pepper and stir well to combine.

7. Add your green beans and white beans to your chicken.

8. Pour in your dressing and toss thoroughly to combine.

9. Serve with a garnish of your mint and enjoy right away.

Recipe 19: Sri Lanka Style Spicy Fish

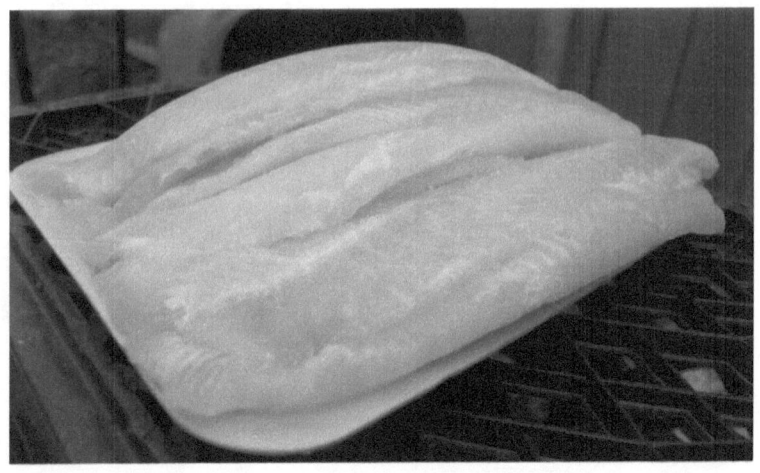

If you are a huge fan of seafood recipes, then this is the perfect dish for you to make. For the tastiest results I highly recommend serving this dish with some healthy veggies or fruits to make this dish truly unique.

Yield: 4 Servings

Preparation Time: 20 Minutes

List of Ingredients:

- 5.2 Ounces of Fish Fillets, White in Color
- 1 Tablespoon of Olive Oil, Extra Virgin Variety
- 3 tablespoons of Spice Mix, Sri Lankan Variety
- 11 Ounces of Couscous, Israeli Variety
- 2 ½ to 3 Cups of Vegetable Stock, Reduced in Sodium Variety
- ¼ Cup of Parsley, Fresh and Roughly Chopped
- ½ of Capsicum, Red in Color and Finely Chopped
- 1 Lemon, Rinded Variety
- 1.8 Ounces of Almonds, Toasted and Flaked
- Some Broccoli, Blanched and for Serving
- Some Wedges of Lemon, For Serving

xxxxxxxxxxxxxxxxxxxxxxxxxxxxxxxxxxxxxxxx

Instructions:

1. The first thing that you will want to do is brush both sides of your fillets with some oil and rub with your spice mix. Set aside for later use.

2. Next cook your couscous according to the directions on the package.

3. Take a medium sized saucepan and bring your stock and oil together. Set over medium heat and bring to a boil. Once boiling cover and remove from heat. Allow to stand for at least 5 minutes.

4. Fluff your couscous after this time.

5. Add in your parsley, lemon rind, almonds and capsicum. Stir thoroughly to combine.

6. Then blanch your broccoli in some water. Drain and set aside for later use.

7. Next cook up your fish. To do this heat up a large sized skillet placed over medium heat. Once your pan is hot enough add in your fish fillets and cook for at least 5 to 10 minutes on each side or until the fish flakes easily with a fork.

8. Remove and serve your fish on top of a bed of couscous, your broccoli and a lemon wedge. Enjoy.

Recipe 20: Roasted Cauliflower with Lemon and Olives

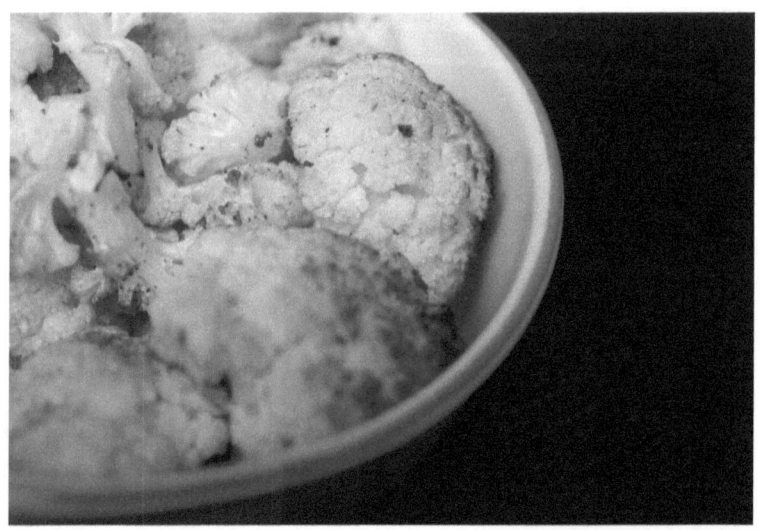

This is one gestational diabetes dish that you are going to love, especially if you love dishes that are just as colorful as the environment outside. This is a dish that contains a minimal number of carbs, making it a diabetic friendly food that you can enjoy during your pregnancy.

Yield: 4 Servings

Preparation Time: 30 Minutes

List of Ingredients:

- 1 Tablespoon of Olive Oil, Extra Virgin Variety
- Some Cooking Spray
- 1 Head of Cauliflower, Cut into Florets
- 1 Tablespoon of Paprika, Powdered and Smoked Variety
- 2 tablespoons of Lemon, Chopped Finely
- ¾ Cup of Black Olives
- 1 Red Capsicum, Large in Size, Roasted and Sliced into Strips
- ½ Cup of Parsley, Fresh and Torn Roughly
- 1 Lemon, Juice Only

XXXXXXXXXXXXXXXXXXXXXXXXXXXXXXXXXXXXXXX

Instructions:

1. The first thing that you will want to do is preheat your oven to 375 degrees.

2. While your oven is heating up coat your cauliflower in paprika until thoroughly coated. Place onto a generously greased baking tray.

3. Spray with some cooking spray and place into your oven to bake for the next 25 minutes, making sure to turn over once.

4. In a large sized bowl and add in your cauliflower, lemon, olives, capsicum, fresh lemon juice, olive oil and parsley.

5. Toss thoroughly to combine and serve right away.

Recipe 21: Tasty Fennel and Almond Salad

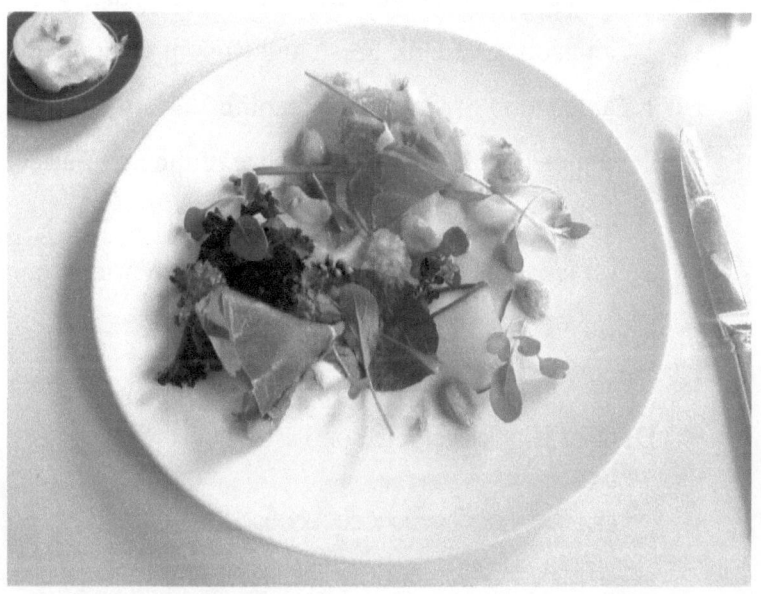

If you are looking for a tasty and light salad to enjoy, you can go wrong with making this dish. The fennel used in this dish helps to add a natural sweetness to this salad dish that I know you are going to fall in love.

Yield: 2 Servings

Preparation Time: 5 Minutes

List of Ingredients:

- 3 tablespoons of Lemon Juice, Fresh
- 2 tablespoons of Olive Oil, Extra Virgin Variety
- 1 Tablespoon of Dill, Fresh and Roughly Chopped
- 1 Tablespoon of Currants, Heaping Variety
- 2 Fennel Bulbs, Medium in Size, Julienne Variety and Thinly Sliced
- 1 Tablespoon of Almonds, Slivered Variety and Lightly Toasted
- 1 Cup of Arugula Leaves, Fresh
- Dash of Black Pepper, For Taste

XXXXXXXXXXXXXXXXXXXXXXXXXXXXXXXXXXXXXXXX

Instructions:

1. The first thing that you will want to do is combine your fresh lemon juice, olive oil, dill and currants in a large sized mixing bowl until evenly mixed together.

2. Add your fennels to your mixing bowl and toss to thoroughly combine.

3. Serve your arugula leaves with a topping of your almonds and your premade dressing.

4. Season with a dash of pepper and enjoy right away.

Recipe 22: Nicoise Style Salad

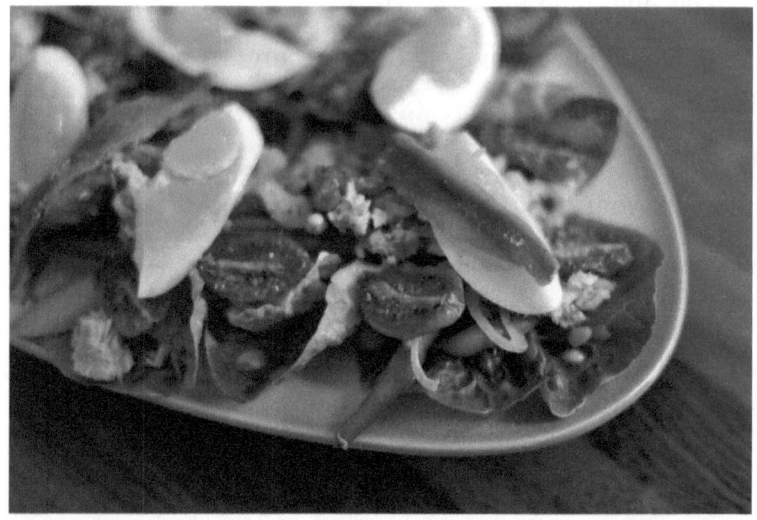

This delicious salad recipe is packed with a variety of different vegetables and flavors that I know you won't be able to get enough of. Feel free to use whatever veggies you wish to make this dish truly delicious.

Yield: 2 Servings

Preparation Time: 12 Servings

List of Ingredients:

- 13 Ounces of Potatoes, New Variety and Small in Size
- 1 Ounce of Green Beans, French Variety and Trimmed
- ½ Pound of Cherry Tomatoes Cut into Halves
- ½ Cup of Olives, Kalamata Variety
- 6 Mushrooms, Button Variety and Thinly Sliced
- 1, 10 Ounce Can of tuna, In Water and Drained
- 1 Tablespoon of Capers, Small in Size and Optional
- ½ Tablespoon of Olive Oil, Extra Virgin Variety and Light
- 1 Tablespoon of Vinegar, Red Wine Variety
- 3 Anchovies, Optional
- 2 Eggs, Hardboiled Variety, Peeled and Cut into Quarters
- 1 Handful of Salad, Your Favorite Kind

xxxxxxxxxxxxxxxxxxxxxxxxxxxxxxxxxxxxxxx

Instructions:

1. Place your potatoes into a large sized saucepan and fill with some cold water. Bring this mixture to a boil over medium heat and cook for the next 7 to 8 minutes or until tender to the touch.

2. During the last two minutes or cooking add in your beans.

3. Then drain and rinse your mixture with some water. Drain for a second time.

4. Cut your potatoes into quarters and add into a large sized bowl.

5. Add in your beans, tomatoes, olives, capers, tuna and mushrooms.

6. Then whisk together your oil, vinegar and anchovies.

7. Season with a dash of salt and pepper.

8. Serve your salad with your dressing over the top. Top off with your egg quarters and enjoy right away.

Recipe 23: Tasty Grilled Salmon

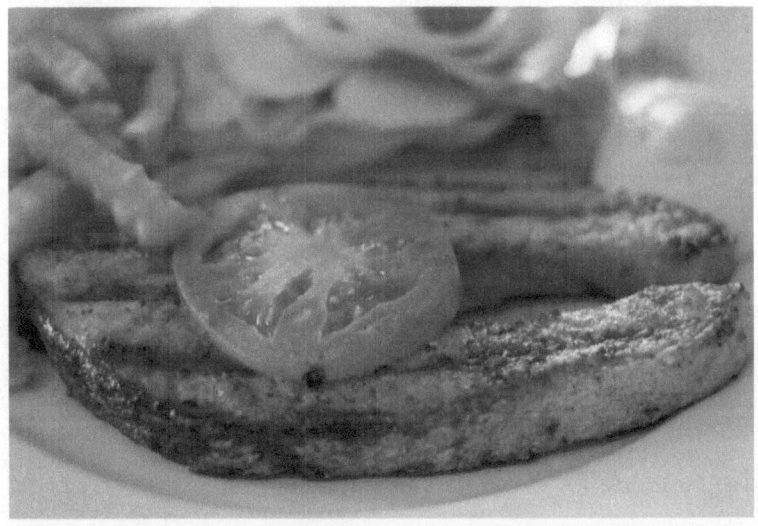

Here is a flexible seafood dish that I know you are going to fall in love with. It is incredibly flexible, making it easy for you to add any of your favorite fruits and veggies to it to make it truly delicious.

Yield: 2 Servings

Preparation Time: 15 Minutes

List of Ingredients:

- Some Cooking Spray
- 2 Salmon Fillets, 5 to 6 Ounces Each
- 2.6 Ounces of Spinach Leaves, Baby Variety, Dried and Washed
- 2 Carrots, Large in Size, Peeled and Cut into Small Sized Sticks
- 7 Ounces of Pasta, Cooked Variety and Risoni Variety

Ingredients for Your Gremolata:

- 1 Bunch of Parsley, Flat Leaf Variety, Wash and Roughly Chopped
- 2 Lemons, Fresh, Zested and Juice Only
- 1 Clove of Garlic, Crushed and Finely Chopped
- 1 Tablespoon of Olive Oil, Extra Virgin Variety
- ¼ teaspoon of Chili, Fresh and Optional

xxxxxxxxxxxxxxxxxxxxxxxxxxxxxxxxxxxxxxxx

Instructions:

1. The first thing that you will want to do is prepare your gremolata first. To do this combine all of your ingredients for your gremolata in a large sized bowl and use a hand blender to mix thoroughly. Set aside for later use.

2. Then lightly grease a large sized skillet placed over medium to high heat.

3. Season your fish with some salt and pepper and place into your skillet to cook for at least 4 minutes on each side or until crispy.

4. Next cook your carrots and risoni according to the directions on the package.

5. Serve your fillets on a bed of fresh spinach and your risoni.

6. Top your dish with your gremolata and your carrots. Enjoy right away.

Recipe 24: Japanese Style Coleslaw

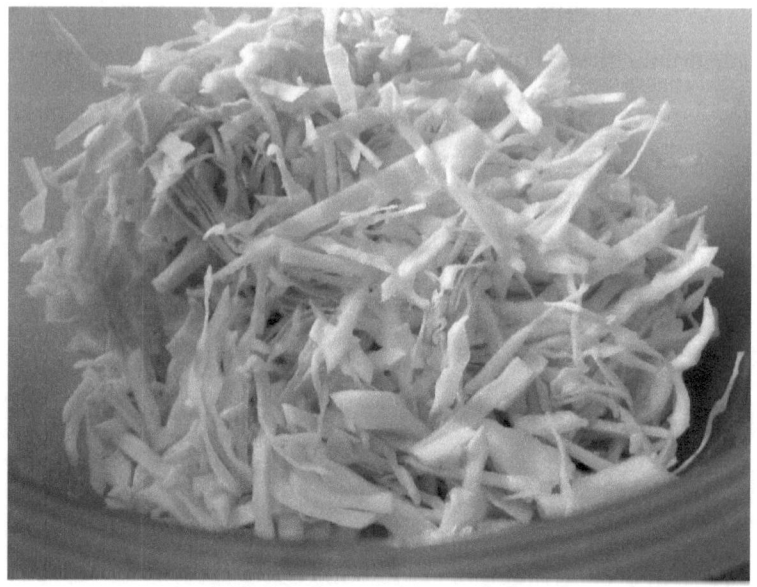

Here is yet another crunchy and sweet tasty side salad that even the pickiest of eaters are going to fall in love with. For the best results I highly recommend serving this dish without your dressing to keep it as crisp as possible.

Yield: 2 Servings

Preparation Time: 10 Minutes

List of Ingredients:

- ¼ of a green Cabbage, Core Remove and Finely Shaved
- 1 Daikon, Small in Size, Julienne Style
- 1 Carrot, Medium in Size and Cut into Julienne Style
- 3 Shallots, Sliced Finely
- ½ Bunch of Coriander, Stems Chopped and Leaves Picked
- 2 tablespoons of Sesame Seeds, Black in Color and Toasted

Ingredients for Your Dressing:

- 1 Tablespoon of Miso Paste
- 1 teaspoon of Tahini
- 1 Tablespoon of Vinegar, Brown Rice Variety
- 1 Tablespoon of Oil, Sesame Variety
- ½ teaspoon of Soy Sauce, Low in Sodium

XXXXXXXXXXXXXXXXXXXXXXXXXXXXXXXXXXXXXXX

Instructions:

1. The first thing that you will want to do is combine your cabbage, daikon and carrots together in a large sized bowl until thoroughly combine.

2. Add in your shallots, coriander and sesame seeds and toss again to combine.

3. Then use a separate mixing bowl and add in all of your ingredients for your dressing into it. Whisk well until evenly combine. Add in at least ½ a tablespoon of water into it to thin it out.

4. Pour over your salad and toss well to combine.

5. Season your salad with your pepper and toss again.

6. Serving right away and enjoy.

Recipe 25: Cumin Spiced Carrots

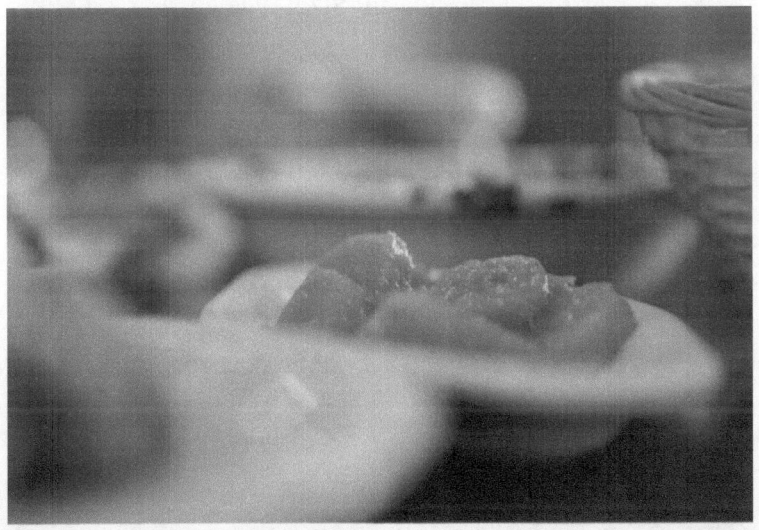

Here is a healthy and delicious vegetable dish that I know you are going to fall in love with. This is a great recipe to make if you are looking for something on the spicy and exotic side.

Yield: 2 Servings

Preparation Time: 5 Minutes

List of Ingredients:

- 4 Carrots, Medium in Size, Peeled and Cut into Halves
- 1 teaspoon of Olive Oil, Extra Virgin Variety
- ¼ Cup of Parsley, Fresh and Roughly Chopped
- 1 teaspoon of Cumin, Ground
- 1 Lemon, Small in Size and Juice Only

xxxxxxxxxxxxxxxxxxxxxxxxxxxxxxxxxxxxx

Instructions:

1. The first thing that you will want to do is cook your carrots in a medium sized saucepan filled with boiling water. Cook your carrots until they are tender to the touch. Once tender remove, drain and set aside for later use.

2. Next return your carrots to your pan and add in your oil, parsley and fresh lemon juice.

3. Toss thoroughly to combine and serve while still warm.

About the Author

Heston Brown is an accomplished chef and successful e-book author from Palo Alto California. After studying cooking at The New England Culinary Institute, Heston stopped briefly in Chicago where he was offered head chef at some of the city's most prestigious restaurants. Brown decide that he missed the rolling hills and sunny weather of California and moved back to his home state to open up his own catering company and give private cooking classes.

Heston lives in California with his beautiful wife of 18 years and his two daughters who also have aspirations to follow in their father's footsteps and pursue careers in the culinary arts. Brown is well known for his delicious fish and chicken dishes and teaches these recipes as well as many others to his students.

When Heston gave up his successful chef position in Chicago and moved back to California, a friend suggested he use the internet to share his recipes with the world and so he did! To date, Heston Brown has written over 1000 e-books that contain recipes, cooking tips, business strategies for catering companies and a self-help book he wrote from personal experience.

He claims his wife has been his inspiration throughout many of his endeavours and continues to be his partner in business as well as life. His greatest joy is having all three women in his life in the kitchen with him cooking their favourite meal while his favourite jazz music plays in the background.

Author's Afterthoughts

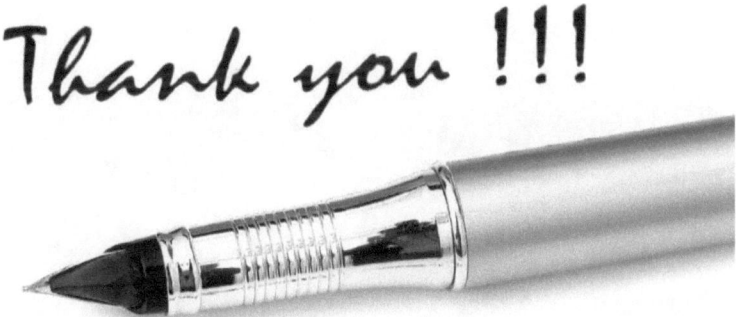

Thank you to all the readers who invested time and money into my book! I cherish every one of you and hope you took the same pleasure in reading it as I did in writing it.

Out of all of the books out there, you chose mine and for that I am truly grateful. It makes the effort worth it when I know my readers are enjoying my work from beginning to end.

Please take a few minutes to write an Amazon review so that others can benefit from your opinions and insight. Your review will help countless other readers make an informed choice

Thank you so much,

Heston Brown

www.ingramcontent.com/pod-product-compliance
Lightning Source LLC
Chambersburg PA
CBHW031235280526
45784CB00004B/1585